Improving Your Memory

Improving Your Memory

How to Remember What You're Starting to Forget

REVISED EDITION

Janet Fogler
and
Lynn Stern

The Johns Hopkins University Press
Baltimore and London

Copyright 1988 Janet Fogler and Lynn Stern
© 1994 The Johns Hopkins University Press
All rights reserved. Published 1994
Printed in the United States of America on acid-free paper

03 02 01 00 99 98 97 96 95 94   5 4 3 2

The Johns Hopkins University Press
2715 North Charles Street
Baltimore, Maryland 21218-4319
The Johns Hopkins Press Ltd., London

ISBN 0-8018-4768-0 (pbk.: alk. paper)

Library of Congress Cataloging-in-Publication Data will be found
at the end of this book.

A catalog record for this book is available from the British Library.

We would like to express our appreciation and gratitude to the W. K. Kellogg Foundation and to all of our colleagues at the University of Michigan Medical Center's Turner Geriatric Services, especially Ruth Campbell. We are also indebted to Bea Wooley and all the Turner Peer Counselors who began the memory program in 1978. Lastly, we want to thank Scott and Neal for their good humor and support.

Contents

Preface   ix

1. **How Memory Works   1**

2. **How Memory Changes as People Age   17**

3. **Factors Affecting Memory for People of All Ages   27**

4. **Memory Improvement Techniques   59**

   General Tips for Remembering   91

   Answers to the Exercises   95

   Recommended Reading   99

Preface

If you frequently say, "I just can't remember anymore!" or "My memory has gotten *so* bad!" you may have given in to the myth that aging and memory loss go hand in hand. In fact, it is the belief in this myth that keeps many people from even *trying* to remember. People of all ages complain about forgetting, but older people often worry about getting "senile" when they cannot remember a cousin's name or where they put their appointment book. There *are* changes in memory as people grow older, but, for almost everyone, memory can be improved with training and practice.

No one can remember everything. People of all ages must make choices about what they want to remember and put effort and energy into those areas that are most important to them. This self-help manual will enable you to make these choices, based on an understanding of how memory works and how it changes with age, and will give you concrete strategies for tackling the areas of memory that trouble you.

In order to make the basic information more meaningful, we have included many examples from everyday life, pen-and-paper exercises demonstrating concepts and techniques, and assignments for applying what you have learned to your daily life.

You will get the most out of this book if you read it carefully, do all of the exercises, and make an effort to use the suggestions in your daily life.

Improving Your Memory

1 How Memory Works

___

To improve the memory process, it helps to understand how memory works. Although the brain is not understood nearly as well as the heart or the circulatory system, memory experts have devised a way to visualize how we remember. They often describe the memory process as consisting of three stages.

The Three Stages of Memory

Sensory memory, the first stage in the memory process, is the very brief recognition by the mind of what the senses take in. We become aware of information through the senses—vision, hearing, touch, smell, and taste. In the world in which we live, we are constantly surrounded by sights and sounds. Much of what the eye sees and the ear hears is discarded immediately. There is no need for us to record it. However, when the sensory impression is paid attention to, it enters the second stage of memory, known as short-term memory.

Short-term memory may be equated with conscious thought—the very small amount of material that you can hold in your mind at any one moment. Most experts believe that short-term memory can hold no more than six or seven items. This material will be forgotten in five to ten seconds, unless it is continually repeated or it is transferred to long-term memory.

An example of information that is held in short-term memory and generally discarded without being stored is a seven-digit telephone number. When you look up a phone number, close the phone book, dial the number, and get a busy signal, you often realize that you've already forgotten the number you just dialed. This is a good demonstration of how briefly information is held in short-term memory. *It is important to keep in mind that not all information that registers in short-term memory gets stored in long-term memory.*

Long-term memory, the memory bank, is the largest component of the memory system. Its storage space is practically limitless. A common misconception is that long-term memory refers to events that occurred a long time ago. In fact, long-term memory holds information that was learned as recently as a few minutes ago and as long ago as many decades. This storage space holds items as varied as:

- your name

- what happened an hour ago

- where you spent last Thanksgiving

- the information needed to drive a car

- the image of your first-grade teacher

- the multiplication tables

Thus, long-term memory refers to any information that is no longer in conscious thought but is stored for potential recollection.

The diagram on page 3 summarizes the memory process, which is more fully explained on the following pages.

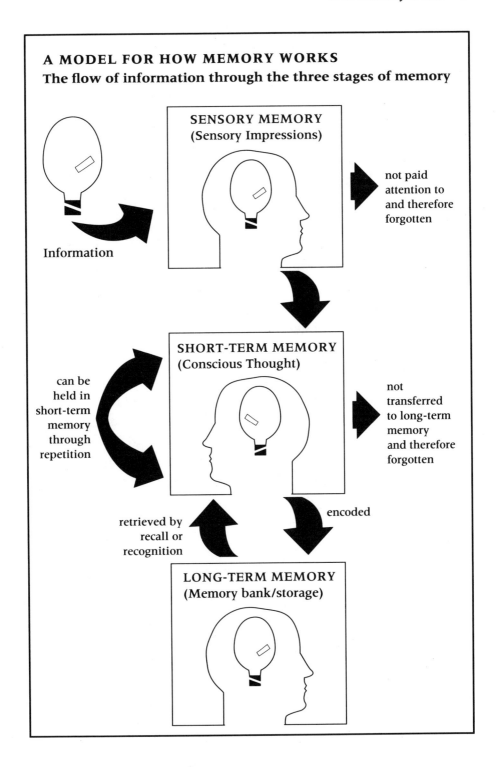

A MODEL FOR HOW MEMORY WORKS
The flow of information through the three stages of memory

SENSORY MEMORY
(Sensory Impressions)

Information

not paid
attention to
and therefore
forgotten

SHORT-TERM MEMORY
(Conscious Thought)

can be
held in
short-term
memory
through
repetition

not
transferred
to long-term
memory
and therefore
forgotten

encoded

retrieved by
recall or
recognition

LONG-TERM MEMORY
(Memory bank/storage)

Here is an example of how the memory process works in daily life.

EXAMPLE

- You are doing your weekly shopping at the local grocery store. There are many items on the shelves which make sensory impressions on you. You see the colors of the packages, smell the bakery products, and hear the many sounds going on around you. However, these *sensory* impressions may or may not register in conscious thought.

- You pause in the produce department and consider what fruit is in season at this time of year. You glance at a papaya, a fruit that you have never tried, and notice that it is very expensive. If you then move on, you will probably not recall the papaya in any detail. The impression of the papaya has entered *short-term memory* or consciousness but has not necessarily been stored in long-term memory.

- However, if you pay more attention to the papaya by noting its shape, color, and texture, smelling its fragrance, feeling its ripeness, and even thinking about what it might taste like or how you could prepare it, you will probably transfer the image and knowledge of that fruit into *long-term memory*. This information will be available for retrieval in the future, for example, when you see a recipe that includes papaya as an ingredient.

Remembering: Encoding and Retrieval

Remembering can be defined as learning and storing information so that it can be retrieved at some future time. Thus, *successful* remembering consists of:

1. getting information solidly into long-term memory (encoding) and
2. retrieving information when it is needed.

Let's discuss what is involved in these two aspects of the process of memory.

Encoding

Researchers use the term *encoding* to describe the process of getting information into long-term memory. Encoding may consist of a number of mental tasks, such as paying attention to something, reasoning it through, associating it with something already known, analyzing it, and elaborating on the details. Often these tasks are performed automatically without any conscious effort on our part. These tasks give deeper meaning to the information and strengthen our chances of remembering it. Perhaps the easiest way to understand encoding is to look at the way it works in everyday life.

EXAMPLES

- Mrs. Yang is a confirmed people-watcher. She loves to sit on a park bench and observe life around her. On any given day, she is aware that there are many people in the park walking their dogs. One day a puppy came up and licked her leg. She petted him, felt his soft fur, and enjoyed his exuberance. She asked the owner the puppy's name and breed. She watched as the puppy explored the riverside area. Several days later when she read her grandson a story about a puppy, she recalled the event and described the puppy in the park to him. She was surprised that she remembered the puppy's name and breed so clearly. Although she had no recollection of the many other dogs she saw that day, the information about the puppy had been well encoded because she had been interested, had paid attention, and had elaborated on the details of the interaction.

- On another day in the park, Mrs. Yang sat next to a friendly woman about her age. After sharing a warm conversation, her new friend introduced herself as Mrs. Meadors. Mrs. Yang thought to herself, "I wish I could remember her name as well as I remember the name of the cute puppy I met." Instead of assuming that she couldn't do it, she decided to give it some thought and see if she could figure out a way to remember it. When she discovered that Mrs. Meadors grew up on a farm, she thought, "I can picture her in a meadow, which sounds like Meadors." In this example, Mrs. Yang intentionally encoded the information by paying attention to it, analyzing it, and associating it with something already known.

Two tasks of encoding—attention and association—deserve some additional emphasis.

Attention.   The first step in the process of encoding information into long-term memory is paying attention. Paying attention is one of the tasks of short-term memory. At any given moment, there are many pieces of information competing for the attention of your short-term memory. It may take some conscious effort on your part to focus your attention on what you need to remember. Keep in mind that the amount of material you can hold in your short-term memory is very limited. You need to zero in on what is important.

EXAMPLES

- A friend tells you to meet her for lunch at 12:00, and you make a note of the date and time in your appointment book. You mistakenly arrive at the restaurant at 12:30 because you didn't pay particular attention when the time was discussed, and you wrote it down incorrectly. Next time, resolve to focus your attention on the details of time and place, and be sure you write them down correctly.

- You were given directions to a new dentist's office and had no trouble finding it the first time. For a second visit, you assume that you will remember where to go. As you approach the area, you realize that you don't know which high-rise building his office is in. What has happened is that you didn't pay enough attention to the location and the appearance of the building. In the future, note some landmarks and descriptive features that will differentiate one building from the next.

In both of these examples the subjects believed that they were paying enough attention to encode the information sufficiently, but clearly they weren't. Everyone has had this experience many times. We give superficial attention to a piece of information and then are frustrated when we can't remember it exactly. One of the simplest ways to improve your memory is to realize the importance of focusing your attention on what you really want to remember. In the future, when you forget, ask yourself if the problem was inadequate attention.

Association. Another aspect of encoding that deserves some explanation is association. Whether we are aware of it or not, new information is encoded by connecting it with other well-known and relevant information that already exists in long-term memory. This process is called association. The easiest way to understand the concept of association is to look at how it happens effortlessly in daily life.

EXAMPLES

• If you meet a new person, your memory of him may be encoded by making a number of different associations. You note what he looks like; where you met him; where he lives; what kind of work he does; and any friends you have in common. Thus an association could be made with these different classifications: curly haired people; the theater where you met him; other people who live in his neighborhood; the medical profession; or the woman who introduced him to you. In the future, thinking of any of these categories could trigger a recollection of your new acquaintance. When you see another curly haired person, or a doctor, or go to the theater, the experience may serve as a cue, and you may think of your new acquaintance.

- Suppose your granddaughter has recently been chosen to be on the high-school field-hockey team. You don't know anything about how the game is played or the equipment that's used. However, you do know something about football. When your granddaughter explains the game and equipment to you, you automatically associate the new information about field size, scoring, timekeeping, and protective equipment with what you already know about football. Without any such associations, information about field hockey would be difficult to encode. The next time you watch football on TV, you may think of your conversation with your granddaughter and remember that she has a field-hockey game coming up.

Much association of new information is done unconsciously, but you can make a conscious effort to associate something you want to remember with something you already know. The more effort you put into creating these associations and the greater the number of cross-references available, the more likely you are to recall at will. In Chapter 4, on memory improvement techniques, we will discuss how you can use association to help you remember.

Retrieval

Retrieval is the process of getting information from long-term memory into the conscious state of short-term memory. Most memory complaints center on the inability to bring to mind information on demand. In actuality, however, our ability to find a piece of information in our vast storehouse of memories and bring it to awareness is truly amazing and happens easily most of the time.

There are two ways by which information you have processed and stored in long-term memory is retrieved.

Recall: a self-initiated search of long-term memory for information

Recognition: perceiving information that is presented to you as something or someone you already know

In most cases recognition is easier than recall. When you say "I can't remember," you usually mean "I can't recall." Even though you cannot recall the name of your representative in Congress, you may easily recognize it when you see it. It may be hard to recall the name of a particular TV show, but you recognize it easily when you see it in the *TV Guide*.

Recall of information is often triggered by a cue. A cue is an event, thought, picture, word, sound, or so forth that triggers the retrieval of information from long-term memory. For example, you may be able to recall the last name of your congressman when prompted with his first name. This triggering information, his first name, is a cue.

People often say, "I can't remember names, but I never forget a face." The reason we remember faces easily is that they present themselves for *recognition*. Remembering names, on the other hand, involves *recall* of information from long-term memory, for which the face is only a cue. When we are searching for a name or other piece of information, we can think of related facts, which may serve as cues, and will often trigger the desired piece of information. For example, if you are having trouble recalling what course you took in summer school, you might think about where it was held, who was in the class with you, and the subjects you have taken in the past.

EXERCISE: RECALL

In order to answer the following questions you are required to recall *the information from long-term memory. If you find this task difficult, try to see if you can* recognize *the correct answers to the questions as they are asked again on p. 13.*

1. What is the name of the hometown of the comic strip character Lil' Abner?

   _____

2. Who played Dorothy in the movie *The Wizard of Oz?*

   _____

3. What is the name of the island in the Pacific Ocean which is famous for a photograph taken of U.S. Marines raising the American flag after a fierce battle with the Japanese?

   _____

4. Who was vice-president of the United States in Richard Nixon's first administration?

   _____

See p. 95 for answers.

Forgetting

It is important to recognize that no one can remember everything. An essential part of the memory process is making decisions about what information is valuable and worth the effort it takes to encode it. Is it really critical to spend energy in encoding the name of a woman who occasionally teaches your exercise class when she is only an infrequent substitute? It might be better to choose to learn the names of your grandson's new wife and her parents.

Most people feel very frustrated and even embarrassed when they have to say, "I've forgotten." However, before you blame a faulty memory, it's important to understand that there are some good reasons for not remembering.

1. *Some information never gets into the memory bank.* It only gets as far as sensory memory or short-term memory. Why? You didn't pay attention to it. You didn't really hear it. You didn't understand it. You didn't care enough to remember it. You got distracted by something else. You didn't need to remember it.

2. *Memories that do enter the memory bank may be overladen with subsequent similar information that makes the original memory irretrievable.* People often describe their inadequacies in memory by saying, "I can't even remember what I ate for breakfast yesterday." If you eat similar types of breakfast food day after day, you may forget what you ate on any particular morning, while the memory of the one time you ate octopus remains firm.

3. *Information for which you have few associations and little background knowledge is harder to remember.* For example, if you are just a beginner at the game of bridge, you will find it hard to remember any particular hand dealt during an evening of play, but a bridge expert can accurately recall all of the cards in a particularly meaningful hand.

4. *Some information may only be remembered when the proper cues are available, and those cues are not part of everyday life.* For example, you may think you've forgotten many of your eighth-grade classmates until you find an old photo or go to a class reunion.

5. *It is believed that some memories fade away.* They are not readily

available for all time. For example, if you studied a foreign language in high school, you may recall or recognize many of the vocabulary words you learned. However, there undoubtedly are many other words you have no recollection of and no longer recognize.

6. *Memories change over time.* A common misconception is that information stored in long-term memory remains stable. If an event is recounted from time to time over a number of years, we are more likely to retain a memory of it; however, the content of the memory is also likely to be changed. As we reflect upon it, we unconsciously reconstruct it based on what has happened to us in the interim. This explains why participants in the same event often have very different recollections of it after time has passed.

Review of Terms

Let's review some of the terms used to describe the memory process.

Sensory: referring to the five senses through which all information enters the brain

Short-term memory: equated with conscious thought, it holds the very small amount of information you can pay attention to at a given moment

Long-term memory: the accumulation of information that is not present in conscious thought but is stored for potential recollection

Encoding: learning and storing information

Retrieval: bringing information from long-term memory to conscious thought

Association: the connection between new information and what you already know

Recall: a self-initiated search of long-term memory for information

Recognition: perceiving information that is presented to you as something or someone you already know

Cue: the event, thought, picture, word, sound, and so on that triggers the retrieval of information from long-term memory

EXERCISE: RECOGNITION

*In order to answer the following questions you are required to
recognize the correct answers.*

1. What is the name of the hometown of the comic strip
    character Lil' Abner?
    Spring Hill
    Dogpatch
    Daisyville

2. Who played Dorothy in the movie *The Wizard of Oz?*
    Doris Day
    Judy Holliday
    Judy Garland

3. What is the name of the island in the Pacific Ocean which is
    famous for a photograph taken of U.S. Marines raising the
    American flag after a fierce battle with the Japanese?
    Oahu
    Iwo Jima
    Guam

4. Who was vice-president of the United States in Richard
    Nixon's first administration?
    John Agnes
    Spiro Agnew
    Gerald Ford

See p. 95 for answers.

EXERCISE: UNDERSTANDING THE MEMORY PROCESS

Complete the blanks in this scenario to test your understanding of the memory process. Use the words listed below.

cue

sensory memory

association

encoding

long-term memory

short-term memory

retrieval

When you go to the library and notice that there are a lot of colorful books on the "new books" shelf, you are using

_____ .

You read through the titles and think about whether they interest you. These conscious thoughts occur in

_____ .

Then you notice a book by a favorite author, James Michener. You take down the book, notice how long it is, read the dust jacket, and decide that you don't have time to read it this month. This process is called

_____ .

The information about the book leaves your conscious thought and goes into

_____ ,

where it may be available for

_____

at another time. When you get home, you notice another of Michener's books in your den. This favorite book serves as a

_____

and reminds you of the book in the library. The connection between the library book and your book is called

_____ .

See p. 95 for answers.

EXERCISE: HOW MEMORY WORKS

True/False. Circle the answer.

T F 1. Short-term memory refers to something that happened within the last two days.

T F 2. All information in conscious thought becomes part of your long-term memory.

T F 3. Sensory impressions may not register in conscious thought.

T F 4. Associations are made both consciously and unconsciously.

T F 5. One piece of new information can be associated with many different facts in your long-term memory.

T F 6. When you are presented with a name that you perceive as something you know, this form of retrieval is called recognition.

T F 7. Once information is encoded in long-term memory, it doesn't change.

See p. 96 for answers.

2 How Memory Changes as People Age

There are many myths about the inevitability of "senility" as people age, but the truth is that the large majority of older people will not face severe memory loss. Sensory memory exhibits little change as people grow older. Older adults usually can register information through their senses in the same way they did when they were younger. The short-term memory capacity is much the same in older and younger people. Thus, an older person experiences little change in her ability to look up an address in her club directory and address an envelope, a task that requires only sensory and short-term memory.

The memory difficulties that most older people describe involve:

Encoding: getting information solidly into long-term memory;
   "I can't remember what I read as well as I used to."

Recall: retrieving information on demand;
   "I know the name of my medicine, but I can't think of it now."

On the other hand, most older people do not describe problems with recognition.

   "I know it when I see it," or "I know it when I hear it."

Although there is considerable variability among all people in terms of memory, many older people can expect changes in the following areas:

Divided attention: It becomes more difficult to pay attention to more than one thing at a time.

Learning new information: It takes greater effort to learn something new.

Retrieval: It is increasingly difficult to access familiar names and vocabulary words on demand.

Recall: It takes longer to recall information from long-term memory.

Accumulation of knowledge: People gain knowledge and wisdom with age.

In this chapter we'll look at each of these five ways that memory changes with age.

It Becomes More Difficult to Pay Attention to More Than One Thing at a Time

As you grow older you may find it harder to attend to two competing activities, thoughts, or conversations. Keep in mind that the amount of information that can be held in short-term memory is very limited, so what you are thinking of can even be displaced by your own new thought. Also, distractions such as a radio playing, someone talking, or a doorbell ringing may disrupt your concentration more now than they used to.

EXAMPLES

• You are in the middle of a discussion at a party when you hear your name mentioned in a nearby conversation. This momentary distraction makes you lose track of what you are saying. You may feel embarrassed and blame your failing memory, but what has actually occurred is that one thought has displaced another in your short-term memory. This is a common experience, and you can simply say," Where was I? I lost my train of thought."

- You have several questions you need to ask your doctor when you see him. When he enters the exam room, you have them well in mind. Then he starts asking you questions about your health. You find that you no longer remember *your* questions. Remembering what you intend to ask your doctor at the same time that you are answering his questions involves a division of attention. If you go to your doctor with a written list of your questions, you will not have to rely on your memory.

EXERCISE: DIVIDED ATTENTION

Can you add this column of figures while you continually repeat the names of the months of the year?

4
8
5
7
<u>9</u>

This exercise demonstrates how difficult it is to pay attention to two fairly simple tasks at one time.

 ASSIGNMENT

During the next few days, notice if your attention is divided while you are trying to read the evening paper or listen to the news. Perhaps the phone rings or you jump up to stir the soup. Maybe your spouse asks you a question. Think about whether these distractions affect your ability to remember what you are reading or listening to. Is it a problem with your memory or are you trying to attend to too many things at once?

It Takes Greater Effort to Learn Something New

Although we know that some information enters long-term memory without effort or awareness, much new learning takes conscious effort and an intent to learn. Too many people believe the myth that "you can't teach an old dog new tricks," but, unless there is impairment of the brain, people can continue to learn and remember throughout life. There are many strategies, some of which will be discussed later in this book, for organizing new information and giving it meaning in order to solidly store it in long-term memory. However, researchers have found that older adults may not spontaneously use the most effective strategies for memory performance. Information that you could learn with little effort in the past may now require greater effort in order to remember. After you decide that it is important for you to remember some new information, you must focus your attention on the task and find some means of encoding the information. As you recall from chapter 1, encoding may include paying attention to something, reasoning it through, analyzing it, associating it with something already known, and elaborating on the details.

EXAMPLE

- Your city council has just enacted new regulations regarding collection of recycled plastic. They will now accept certain plastic containers at curbside, while others are unacceptable. You regularly use, and would like to recycle, detergent, bleach, milk, cottage cheese, and yogurt containers. Because you keep forgetting which items are acceptable, you end up throwing them all in the trash. You decide that you want to easily remember which items to recycle without looking up the regulations each time or asking your neighbor. The first step in learning this new information is giving your undivided attention to reading the information leaflet from the recycling center. You focus on the portion that describes what to do with plastics. The next step is thinking about how you can remember which of your commonly collected plastic items can go in the recycling bin. You note that the milk, bleach, and detergent containers are acceptable, whereas the cottage cheese and yogurt containers are not. After analyzing the situation, you realize that the three acceptable plastic items all contain liquids, whereas the others contain solids. Grouping these containers into other classifications, such as color, size, or shape, might also produce a solution to your problem. You could easily have said, "It's too complicated for me. I can't remember all these distinctions." Instead you decided that it was important to learn and found a means of encoding the information.

EXERCISE: LEARNING NEW INFORMATION

Here is some new information for you to learn and remember. Give it your undivided attention and see how much effort it requires for you to answer the questions that follow the reading. Even though the particular subject may not interest you, the challenge is to find a way to remember the material even if it takes greater effort than you thought it would.

Social Network Size Matters, Jobs Study Shows

For older people seeking work, a University of Southern California research team suggests that a key factor in landing a job is not only who you know, but how many. The more relatives and friends older job-seekers had, the study found, the more likely they were to find work.

The researchers, led by assistant professor of social work Michal Mor-Barak, Ph.D., interviewed 146 Los Angeles–area men and women 55 and older who a year earlier had signed up at various public-service agencies for help in finding work. All had retired, lost their jobs, or were trying to re-enter the workforce for reasons ranging from financial need to boredom. The study found that 64 percent got jobs.

Besides social network size, other factors predicting success at finding work were high motivation and a low number of major life changes such as divorce, marriage, death of a family member or close friend.

Half of those surveyed were white, half roughly equal numbers of Hispanics, blacks and Asians. They were better educated than the general population: 40 percent had attended college: 24 percent had degrees, and some of those had advanced degrees.

The study concluded that it's important for older job-seekers to get connected. One route is via a support group, where they can learn from others' experiences and discuss ways to deal with obstacles such as age discrimination.

(Reprinted with permission from *Modern Maturity*. Copyright 1992, American Association of Retired Persons.)

1. What are the most important factors in finding a job?

2. Name another key factor in finding work.

3. Did more than half of the 146 people surveyed find jobs?

4. What is one conclusion of the study?

See p. 96 for answers.

It Is Increasingly Difficult to Access Familiar
Names and Vocabulary Words on Demand

Everyone knows the experience of being halted in mid-sentence when the desired word or name does not immediately spring to mind. The feeling of the word being on the tip of your tongue occurs more frequently as you age. The frustration of this experience can make you feel anxious, and this anxiety further blocks the recall process.

EXAMPLES

- You begin to tell a friend about the movie you saw last night and you're astonished and embarrassed to discover that the title has escaped you. The more irritated you become, the less likely you are to be able to come up with the name. Instead of giving yourself time and cues to retrieve the name of the movie from long-term memory, you find your attention focused on the frustration of forgetting. If you relax and are patient, the information will often come to you.

- You start to tell a friend about the new bird feeder that you put up. "I saw a beautiful cardinal at the bird feeder on my . . ." At that moment the word "porch" escapes you, and you get flustered and say "the outside of my living room." This is a common occurrence that happens to everyone but is experienced more frequently as you grow older.

The next time you find yourself searching for a needed name or word, try to relax, take a deep breath, and see if you can access the information by thinking of related items. If you are still unable to retrieve that needed word, don't fret. It will undoubtedly come to you unbidden while you are thinking of something else.

It Takes Longer to Recall Information from Long-Term Memory

Studies have shown that older adults take more time to recall needed information from long-term memory than younger people. When older adults are given increased time to complete a test, their performances are greatly improved. In untimed tests of recall, older adults perform comparably to younger ones. Keep this in mind when you are impatient with yourself because you don't recall something immediately. Give yourself a little additional time and see if you can come up with the desired information.

EXAMPLE

- Mrs. Chen was given a video recorder for her birthday. She read the instruction manual and learned to follow the steps for its use. She taped her favorite shows regularly for several weeks and felt confident in her ability to record the programs she wanted. When she returned from a two-week trip to visit her son in New Jersey, she began to tape a show on cooking. She was frustrated to discover that she was unable to either recall the steps or find the instruction manual. She decided to give it one more try. As she held the remote control in her hand and tried to think back to her prevacation routine, the steps came back to her bit by bit. She thought to herself, "I'm so glad I didn't give up because I couldn't remember right away."

Expertise and familiarity often more than compensate in a specific area for the slowing down of recall. For example, a seventy-year-old crossword-puzzle buff, who spends some time every day in this endeavor, may be able to recall words commonly needed in crossword puzzles as quickly as or more quickly than most younger people.

People Gain Knowledge and Wisdom with Age

World knowledge, which is defined as a pool of information acquired over a lifetime from both educational and everyday experiences, accumulates with age. In tests that measure knowledge and vocabulary, older adults do as well as or better than younger people. The experiences of a long and rich life can produce a wisdom that young people can only hope to obtain. Memory and experience are the basis of wisdom. Although it takes greater effort to learn something new, older adults have the wisdom to determine what new information is important to them.

EXERCISE: HOW MEMORY CHANGES

True/False. Circle the answer.

T   F   1. There is no escaping "senility" as you grow older.

T   F   2. If you have always been able to do several things at once, age won't affect this ability.

T   F   3. Sensory and short-term memory exhibit little change as people grow older.

T   F   4. Older adults take longer to recall information from long-term memory.

T   F   5. Older adults spontaneously use memory strategies more often than younger adults.

T   F   6. One way to access well-known information when you can't recall it is to provide yourself with cues by thinking of related items.

See p. 96 for answers.

3 Factors Affecting Memory for People of All Ages

It is known that certain factors can affect the memory process for people of all ages. However, the impact of these factors is likely to be greater as you age, because older people often experience more of these negative influences at one time. We have identified the following factors that commonly affect memory:

- problems with attention
- negative expectations
- stress
- anxiety
- depression
- loss and grief
- inactivity
- lack of organization in daily life
- fatigue
- some physical illnesses
- some medications
- vision and hearing problems
- alcohol
- poor nutrition

As you read through this section, think about which of these factors might be affecting your memory. Awareness of possible causes of memory problems can lead to solutions.

Problems with Attention

Inadequate Attention

In the discussion of how memory works in Chapter 1, we emphasized the importance of focusing attention on what you want to remember. If you really want to remember something, paying adequate attention is the first step. Here are some examples where inadequate attention affected the encoding of new information.

EXAMPLES

- Connie may be daydreaming when her husband asks her to pick up the dry cleaning. Later, when he asks for his suit, she doesn't even remember the request.

- A new resident of Brad's apartment building, Jane Blair, meets him at the mailboxes and introduces herself. He greets her by name and begins a friendly conversation. When they are joined by another resident a few minutes later, Brad discovers that he has no recollection of Jane's name.

The problem in these two examples is that Connie and Brad have not paid enough attention to encoding the needed information so that they can recall it. Paying adequate attention to details can eliminate some instances of forgetting. Ask yourself, "When is it really important for me to pay attention?" At these times, resolve to focus your awareness on the task or information at hand.

Distractions

As you recall from chapter 1, paying attention is one of the tasks of short-term memory. It is important to remember that the amount of information that can be held in your short-term memory is very limited. Any new sound, sight, or thought may distract you and displace what is currently in your short-term memory.

EXAMPLES

- You are certain to have had the experience of going into another room and forgetting what you went for. As you went into the kitchen to get the scissors, perhaps you thought, "I wonder if the mail is here." This new thought replaced the thought of the scissors you needed from the kitchen.

- When you leave your umbrella in the doctor's office, it may be because you are thinking of getting your prescription filled before the drugstore closes.

- You're driving to a movie with a friend. Her conversation draws your attention from noticing exactly where you are, and you forget to get into the left turn lane until it's too late. To avoid this frustrating experience, you might want to ask your passenger to hold her conversation until you get to the movie theater.

These experiences are familiar to people of all ages, but keep in mind that older adults find it more difficult to pay attention to more than one thing at a time. Rather than thinking you can do nothing about these frustrating experiences, try to recognize the limitations of short-term memory and cut out distractions when possible. It is especially important to give your undivided attention to situations that could be potentially dangerous, such as driving, cooking, and taking medications.

EXERCISE: DISTRACTIONS

Below are two short articles. Read the first one in a quiet room, and then read the second one with some competition for your attention, such as the TV or radio.

Fabulous Fakery

Chang Dai-chien, with his floor-length robes, 11th century scholar's cap and four wives (at the same time), cut a striking figure wherever he went. He also attracted much interest as one of the foremost Chinese painters of the 20th century and a skilled forger of ancient masterpieces (he called them "honest copies"). Chang completed almost 30,000 works over a 60-year career that ended with his death in 1983 at the age of 84. A number of Chang's forgeries can be found in collections in the British Museum, Metropolitan Museum of Art and museums throughout China. A retrospective of 87 of his works will be on display at the St. Louis Art Museum (314-721-0072) August 28–October 25.

Ironwoman

Agnes Reinhard, 66, has run many races along Lake Michigan. "Afterward I'd always want to jump in the lake," she says. She gets her wish when she competes August 16 in the Danskin Women's Triathlon Series presented by BMW in Milwaukee—except she jumps in the lake first for a .75K swim, then rides a bike for 20K, and finishes with a 5K run. Reinhard, of West Allis, Wisconsin, placed first in her age division (60-plus) in last year's triathlon and hopes to do as well this year. A personal best to beat? "I don't worry about time," she says. "I compete for the fun of it." More than 7,500 women are expected to enter the Danskin series, the world's only all-women triathlon, which travels to six U.S. cities and Germany.

(Reprinted with permission from *Modern Maturity.* Copyright 1992, American Association of Retired Persons.)

Did you notice a difference in your ability to remember the details?

Negative Expectations

Compared to younger people, older adults are more pessimistic about their *ability* to remember. Older people often say, "I just can't remember anything anymore," whereas younger people attribute forgetting to a lack of *effort*. When you expect that you are going to fail at something, that expectation is likely to increase the possibility of failure. Negative expectations about memory are likely to cause older people to

- put less effort into remembering
- avoid tasks that require memory
- feel anxious when their memories are tested in daily life

EXAMPLE

- Mrs. Martin recently attended a volunteer appreciation banquet. Although she recognized many faces, she felt embarrassed and anxious when she could not address people by name. She thought, "I can't remember names anymore!" Since that time Mrs. Martin has avoided attending gatherings when she doesn't know everyone extremely well. Although her son-in-law gave her a book on how to remember names, she is sure that those techniques are not useful for someone of her age. She stated this belief to her neighbor, who said that she's had the same experience of forgetting familiar names and found a solution. She keeps lists of names of people who are likely to attend various group functions. Before she attends a function, she reviews the appropriate list, visualizing each person. Mrs. Martin agrees to give this technique a try. She is surprised to find that, if she puts enough effort into it, she is able to remember many of the names. She now has more positive expectations about her ability to remember and no longer avoids situations where memory is required. (In chapter 4, you will learn more about remembering names.)

When you are faced with a task of memory, do you find yourself saying, "I'll never be able to do this. What's the use of trying?" Sometimes we give ourselves negative messages without being aware of it. Be conscious of your self-defeating thoughts about your ability to remember. Substitute this thought: "I'm not sure this will work, but I'll give it a good try."

Stress

When you are feeling stressed, anxious, pressured, or rushed, it is often impossible to:

- pay adequate attention to learning new information
- concentrate on the details you want to recall
- relax long enough to let a memory surface

You are more likely to forget things when you are under major stress—due to factors such as moving, illness, loss, your own retirement or the retirement of your spouse—or even when you are under minor stress caused by experiences such as being late to an appointment, losing your house keys, preparing for company, or seeing your doctor. It is important to realize that you may forget more frequently at times like these and that your memory usually improves as the stress is reduced. When you add worry about forgetting to other stresses, you often increase forgetfulness.

EXAMPLE

- You have been extremely busy all week getting ready for a visit from your son and his family, who live in California. The sink becomes clogged, and the plumber is only available during the time when you are picking up the family from the airport. You arrange to leave a key with a neighbor so that the work can be done. To your horror, you forget to leave the key when you go to the airport. You are stressed, overloaded, and rushing. Thus you forgot to do what you wanted to do most. In a case like this, it's best to do what you need to do before doing anything else. Leave the key the moment you think of it.

Anxiety

Anxiety is characterized as inner distress accompanied by physical symptoms and vague fears. Many people who are highly anxious are unable to focus on anything outside of themselves. Their minds are so filled with worries that they cannot pay attention to external happenings, and their memory failures affect their daily functioning.

Some symptoms of anxiety are:

- nervousness, worry, or fear
- apprehension or a sense of imminent doom
- panic spells
- difficulty concentrating
- insomnia
- fear of potential physical illnesses
- heart pounding or racing
- upset stomach or diarrhea
- sweating
- dizziness or light-headedness
- restlessness or jumpiness
- irritability

EXAMPLE

- Eva describes herself as someone who has always been a worrier, but it has gotten worse as she has grown older. She worries about her high blood pressure, her unmarried son, her granddaughter's thumb-sucking, and her arthritis, which could affect her ability to take care of her home. She has butterflies in her stomach; she doesn't sleep well; she spends most of the day worrying; and she is unable to remember things very well. When she is in the clinic to get a blood pressure reading, she mentions her anxiety to the nurse, who suggests that she should discuss it with the doctor. Dr. Persky recommends a cognitive therapy group for people who are anxious or depressed, where she might learn new ways of dealing with her anxiety and benefit from the group support. In the group,

Eva recognizes that she has no control over her son's unmarried state and her granddaughter's thumb-sucking. She is able to take them off her worry list. The group helps her consider some options for the future in case she is unable to take care of her home. Eva knows that she will continue to be a worrier; however, when she realized the uselessness of worrying about those things that she cannot control and began to make plans for her future, some of her symptoms of anxiety were alleviated, including her memory problems.

Depression

Everyone feels blue off and on during a lifetime. However, ongoing depression is not normal and can affect memory. Older people are not necessarily more prone to depression than younger people, but the losses and physical illnesses that frequently accompany old age can rob the older person of the hope of a better future. Some symptoms of depression are:

- appetite change (decrease in appetite is most common)
- sleep disturbance
- fatigue
- anxiety, fearfulness, excessive worrying
- feelings of hopelessness, helplessness
- decreased concentration, difficulty with memory
- difficulty making decisions
- restlessness, pacing
- irritability
- feeling that life is not worth living
- feeling that nothing gives you pleasure
- feeling sick or tired all the time
- sad mood
- suicidal thoughts

How does depression affect memory?

Motivation: When you are depressed you don't care about remembering your new neighbor's name, the time of your exercise class, or who's running for city council. None of these things seems important.

Concentration: Even if you want to remember how to fill out your Medicare form, depression can make you feel foggy and unable to focus on the task.

Perception: If you are depressed you may view a few instances of forgetting as a sign that you can't remember anything at all.

EXAMPLE

- Mr. McIntyre has experienced bouts of depression for several years. His friends and family noticed that when he was feeling depressed, he forgot appointments, confused the names of his grandchildren, and couldn't remember what happened the day before. The first few times this occurred, his family wondered if he were getting "senile," but, over time, they noticed that when his depression lifted, his memory improved. Thus, Mr. McIntyre and his family recognized that his memory loss was connected to his depression and probably did not indicate progressive deterioration. Rather than accept depression as a normal part of aging, the family encouraged Mr. McIntyre to see his physician for an evaluation. Dr. Smith recommended that the depression be treated by a combination of medication and counseling. He also suggested that, until Mr. McIntyre's depression improved, he should use as many memory aids as possible.

Loss and Grief

When you have experienced a significant loss, you are often overwhelmed with feelings of pain and sadness. It is difficult to focus on anything outside of yourself, and your ability to concentrate is diminished. Memory problems frequently accompany grief and will lessen over time unless the mourner becomes severely depressed.

When we talk about loss and grief, most people think primarily of death. In fact, a feeling of loss may accompany many different experiences, including moving, major surgery, retirement of yourself or your spouse, vision or hearing impairment, illness of a friend or family member, changes in financial circumstances, death of a pet, marriage of a child or friend, and changes in your own health. When two or more of these experiences occur at once, the impact is greatly increased.

EXAMPLES

- Mrs. Hammerman moved into a senior citizens' building after a two-year wait. She had been looking forward to having less responsibility and meeting new people but was surprised at how often she longed for her old home and neighbors. At the same time, she found herself forgetting appointments and family birthdays. She became more and more worried and finally went to see her doctor. After doing some tests, the doctor assured her that she wasn't losing her memory. He explained to Mrs. Hammerman that even a move you want to make may cause a lot of sadness, which can temporarily affect your memory.

- Mr. Miller had been ready to retire for several years when the day finally arrived. He looked forward to sleeping late, having no boss to answer to, and spending time in his basement workshop. However, he was surprised to discover that he often felt sad and at loose ends. He also noticed that he was forgetting things. With his wife's encouragement, he volunteered to deliver Meals on Wheels to shut-ins and began a drawing class. As he felt more useful, his sadness diminished, along with much of his forgetfulness.

Inactivity

Lack of Mental Stimulation

The old adage "Use it or lose it" is often applied to memory functioning. Although the evidence is not all in, keeping mentally active and using memory skills may enhance your ability to remember. Some examples of mental stimulation include:

- attending an adult education class
- participating in a discussion group
- doing crossword puzzles
- playing bridge, chess, or Trivial Pursuit
- answering "Jeopardy" or other quiz show questions
- learning to use a computer
- reading a challenging book
- using newly learned memory techniques

EXAMPLE

- Mrs. Parker has always had a great interest in current events. Although she reads the newspaper daily, she has lately found it difficult to retain the information needed to formulate her position on issues. Rather than give up, she joins the current events discussion group in her senior apartment building. She enjoys the lively discussions and finds that her memory for issues is reinforced by preparing for the group and hearing the opinions of others.

Lack of Social Interaction

Many people agree that social involvement is a major factor in maintaining or improving mental capacities. When days are uncommitted and unstructured, there is less incentive to focus and organize your thoughts, and less need to remember. In social contact you have the opportunity to talk about the week's events, which reinforces the memory of what you have done and learned.

- You receive a letter from your daughter telling you that your granddaughter is running for class president. When your daughter calls later in the week and says, "Jenny won!" you have no idea what she is talking about. Before you assume that your memory is failing, consider the fact that you saw very few people over the week and told no one about the news. If you tell a friend about any new information you receive, you encode it more deeply and greatly increase your chances of remembering it. You have not only used more senses when talking about it (hearing and speaking the words) but also have reinforced the content by discussing it.

- You've been sick for the last month and have hardly left the house. You can't remember much about what happened yesterday or the day before. You're afraid that your memory is failing along with your health. Friends have been trying to get you to go out, but you just haven't felt like it. Finally one day you give in and go to the senior center. You discuss mutual acquaintances and the Detroit Tigers' chances of winning the World Series. These discussions give you something new to think about and trigger old memories you thought you'd forgotten. When you return home, you realize that you haven't been making an effort to learn and remember something new because every day has been the same.

Lack of Physical Activity

Although researchers are currently investigating the connection between physical activity and memory, there is no evidence at this point that you can improve your memory through exercise. However, we know that exercise and other forms of physical activity influence factors that contribute to enhanced longevity, health, and fitness in older adults. As further research is done, we will learn more about the connection between physical activity and mental functioning.

Lack of Organization in Daily Life

Many instances of forgetting and losing things can be traced to a disorganized lifestyle. When you don't have a systematic way to keep track of your appointments, return things to their correct places in your home, pay bills, or store important papers in a safe place, you are more likely to be forgetful. Many people have developed a lifelong habit of being organized, while others are disorganized and have never been bothered by it. If you think that some of your instances of forgetting are due to a lack of organization, you may want to develop some new organizational habits.

EXAMPLES

- Miss Woodring complained, "I always write things down. I know about keeping lists, but then I can't find the lists." At a memory course at her senior center, she heard other participants describe the same situation. The teacher advised them to keep all lists of things to buy or do in one convenient place. Miss Woodring realized she had been making lists on odd scraps of paper and leaving them all over the house. She remedied the situation by keeping a notebook for lists on her kitchen table.

- You get a notice that your electricity is about to be turned off. You're positive that you paid the bills, but when you look in the checkbook there is no record of payment. After searching the house, you discover one bill in a kitchen drawer and another in a book you're reading. No wonder you forgot to pay the bills! Most people can't keep track of household finances without some organized system. When your bills are scattered throughout the house and you have no regular schedule for paying them, it's very easy to neglect one.

✎   ASSIGNMENT ━━━━━━━━━━━━━━━━━━━━━━━━━━━━━

Choose one *area of your life in which you think getting organized will help you remember.*

_____ Keeping track of my purse/keys/glasses/ _____ .

_____ Remembering everything I want at the grocery store.

_____ Remembering to send birthday cards to family and friends.

_____ Remembering to pay my bills on time.

_____ Keeping track of the scissors/tape/pencil sharpener/wrapping paper/ _____ .

_____ Remembering to put gas in the car before it's nearly empty.

_____ Remembering to put the garbage out.

_____ Your choice _____ .

Now that you have chosen one, think of a way that you can organize this area of your life so that you will remember. For example, you might put up a hook where you will always *hang your keys.*

The problem: _____

_____

_____

_____

_____

Your solution: _____

_____

_____

_____

The results: _____

_____

_____

_____

After you have accomplished this goal, why not choose another?

The problem: _____

_____

_____

_____

Your solution: _____

_____

_____

_____

The results: _____

_____

_____

_____

Fatigue

Fatigue affects your ability to concentrate and slows down the recall process. You are more likely to have trouble learning new information when you're tired. Each person should figure out which times of the day he or she is most alert and should do tasks that involve new learning at those times.

EXAMPLES

- You usually read at bedtime because it puts you to sleep. However, you can't keep the characters straight in the book you're reading, and this frustrates you. You might try reading this book when you are more alert. If you want to read before dozing off, read something you don't care about remembering.

- You have just finished the third lecture of a six-week series on health problems. You were especially looking forward to last week's lecture on diabetes because your husband has diabetes in his family. However, you realize that you remember little of the material, because you were especially tired that day. For the next lecture, you resolve to be rested and ready to take notes.

Some Physical Illnesses

Even though most older people do not develop severe memory loss, memory problems can be a sign that the body is not functioning properly. Some of the following physical illnesses can aggravate an already existing mild memory problem, or they can cause memory changes in a person who has previously exhibited no memory loss. Treatment of these conditions can result in partial or complete improvement of memory function.

- infection
- fever
- heart disease

- lung disease
- thyroid problems
- circulatory problems
- liver and kidney problems
- strokes
- dehydration
- low blood sugar
- diabetes
- Parkinson's disease
- anemia
- delirium

On the other hand, some types of diseases or injuries that cause damage to the brain may not be reversible. Alzheimer's disease is the major cause of irreversible memory loss (see Appendix A, p. 51). Strokes and traumatic injury to the head often cause memory problems that show improvement over time but frequently leave some irreversible changes.

If you are concerned about your memory and want to rule out a physical cause, the first step is to see your family doctor, who is familiar with your medical history. However, some physicians receive little training in assessing the mental status of older people. Therefore, it may be worthwhile to consult a physician with specific training in geriatrics who has the diagnostic skills to distinguish among a wide assortment of possible causes of memory loss. A medical assessment often includes:

- a social and medical history taken from both the patient and a relative or friend
- a thorough physical examination
- a neuropsychological exam, which is a series of tests that provide information about the thought processes
- blood tests, which are used to detect thyroid, kidney, and liver malfunctions; certain nutritional deficiencies, such as pernicious anemia or vitamin B12 deficiency; infections; and metabolic and chemical imbalances
- urinalysis, which is used to detect infections

Other possible tests that may be indicated include:

- CT scan (computerized axial tomogram): a special x-ray of the brain
- MRI (magnetic resonance imaging): a procedure that painlessly scans the brain and other body parts using no radiation
- EEG (electroencephalogram): a measurement of electrical activity (brain waves) in the brain
- lumbar puncture (spinal tap): an analysis of spinal fluid that can detect malignancies, neurosyphilis, and certain infections

---
EXAMPLE

- When Cathy, the house cleaner, arrived at Mrs. Thompson's apartment for her weekly visit, she found Mrs. Thompson in bed and quite confused. When Cathy asked her if she had had breakfast, Mrs. Thompson said she wasn't sure. Also, she could not remember Cathy's name or exactly why Cathy was there. Since Mrs. Thompson had never been so confused in the past, Cathy called a neighbor, who decided that Mrs. Thompson should go to the emergency room. The physicians at the hospital discovered that she had a serious urinary tract infection and admitted her to the hospital. When Mrs. Thompson's infection cleared up, her confusion disappeared, and she returned home feeling mentally and physically well.

For more information on Alzheimer's disease, see p. 51.

Some Medications

Some medications can make you feel drowsy or unfocused. They can slow down your recall and make it hard to concentrate. Many older people are taking too many medications or are incorrectly taking what has been prescribed. Both prescription and nonprescription medications can be the cause of confusion or the source of a memory problem. It's important to ask your doctor or pharmacist about all of your medications and their side effects. Also make sure that you keep a record of every medication you are currently taking and keep all medical professionals, including your pharmacist, advised of this record.

Usually confusion or a memory problem develops within a couple of days after a person starts to take a medication, but sometimes these problems occur with a medication that has been taken for a long time. Because the brain of an older person is more sensitive to the chemicals in medications, even a previously well tolerated medication may cause problems. Any time there is a memory problem or confusion, medicines should be considered as possible causes. If the medication is the source of the problem, the confusion or memory problem will improve after the person has stopped taking the medication—usually over several days, though for some medicines the full improvement may take several months. However, a person should stop taking a prescription medicine only if a doctor advises that action.

No one can predict who will experience this type of bad effect from a medication. Memory problems or confusion may be caused by just one drug or by the combination of several. The people most at risk for memory problems from medicines are those with low body weight, those who have had a sudden change in health, those taking many medicines, those with a history of drug allergies, and those with a decrease in kidney or liver function. (This section is adapted from "Medications Causing Confusion," by Leslie Shimp, B.S., Pharm. D., Associate Professor of Pharmacy, University of Michigan, Ann Arbor, Michigan.)

EXAMPLE

- Mr. Romano has been feeling quite tired, a bit foggy, and forgetting more than he used to. His neighbor suggests that he see his family doctor for consultation. Dr. Brown takes a complete history, including a review of medications. She discovers that Mr. Romano has begun to take over-the-counter antihistamines to control his seasonal allergies, along with the sleeping pills that she had prescribed at the last visit. Dr. Brown recognizes that the combination of the two drugs may be causing Mr. Romano's fatigue and memory problems. She prescribes a shorter acting sleeping pill, so that this medication will be out of Mr. Romano's system during the daytime. She also substitutes a nonsedating allergy medication for the antihistamine. Mr. Romano finds that, over time, his memory improves with this combination of medications.

Vision and Hearing Problems

An older person with vision or hearing problems often blames his memory if he can't recall information or experiences. In fact, the problem may not be in the memory at all. When the visual impression is not seen well or the sound is not heard clearly, the information will not be recorded correctly. It is important to admit when you can't see or hear adequately and ask others to speak up or make themselves and their material visible. Frequent vision and auditory testing is necessary to insure that you're getting the aids you need. Vision and hearing abilities can change dramatically, and new technology is continually being developed that may compensate for losses.

EXAMPLES

- Your neighbor suggests that you call a realtor whose name is Abbott. When you call the realty company, you ask for Mr. Babcock. The problem here may not be your memory; your neighbor may have mumbled, or you may have trouble hearing. If you want to remember something correctly, ask the person to repeat it, spell it, or even write it down.

- At the doctor's office, the receptionist gives you an insurance form to complete at home. "Just sign in these three places, and mail it off," she says, pointing to three blanks. When you get home, you are confused by all the blank spaces and say, "I've already forgotten what she told me." However, the problem may not be in your memory. You may not have seen the spaces she pointed to. Next time, ask her to mark the spaces with a red *X*.

Alcohol

Alcohol can affect your memory in two different ways: First, many people find that they are less able to tolerate alcohol as they grow older; two drinks may have been tolerated well in the past but are now too much. The effects of alcohol are more dependent on the amount consumed in one drinking occasion than on how often a person takes a drink. As far as memory is concerned, there is a greater effect on the brain if you have four drinks in one night than if you have one drink on each of four nights. Second, long-term abuse of alcohol can cause irreversible memory loss.

In addition to the direct effects of alcohol on memory, alcohol consumption can cause or worsen other factors that affect your memory:

- Depression: Alcohol acts as a depressant on the central nervous system.
- Nutritional status: Alcohol provides calories without nutritional content. Some people who drink excessively fail to eat an adequate diet.

Poor Nutrition

There is still a great deal to be learned about how nutrition affects memory, but we know that a well-balanced diet contributes to overall health. Some older people eat a limited range of foods, such as toast and canned soup, a diet that can lead to a deficiency of needed nutrients. Fresh fruits and vegetables, whole-grain cereals and breads, and low-fat dairy foods or meat should be eaten daily. Small, frequent meals can be easier to prepare than traditionally larger meals and result in healthier eating habits and adequate intake of calories. Maintaining the appropriate body weight for height and age is especially important. Being either underweight or overweight can be physiologically taxing.

The use of a normal dosage multivitamin supplement is safe and appropriate if the reasons for the inadequate diet are not easily remedied. Megadoses of vitamins or minerals are not safe and should not be taken unless prescribed by a health care provider.

Older adults have increased sensitivity to caffeine, nicotine, and alcohol. They should be used in moderation or avoided altogether.

Community nutrition programs can help older adults maintain healthy eating habits. Eating with others is a very important part of mealtime for many people. Many cities and towns have programs for seniors that offer meals and fellowship in communal settings. Outreach programs can take older adults shopping for food, and homemaker services can help prepare meals in the home. For those who are homebound, there are programs that deliver meals to older adults, such as Meals on Wheels. (Courtesy of nutrition consultant Kate Jones Share, M.S., Clinical Nutritionist.)

For a nutrition checklist, see p. 55.

✎   ASSIGNMENT ━━━━━━━━━━━━━━━━━━━━━━━━━━━

Now that we've explained how different factors affect memory, you can evaluate which factors might be affecting you.

	Never	Sometimes	Always
1. Problems with attention	_____	_____	_____
2. Negative expectations	_____	_____	_____
3. Stress	_____	_____	_____
4. Anxiety	_____	_____	_____
5. Depression	_____	_____	_____
6. Loss and grief	_____	_____	_____
7. Inactivity	_____	_____	_____
8. Lack of organization	_____	_____	_____
9. Fatigue	_____	_____	_____
10. Physical illness	_____	_____	_____
11. Medication	_____	_____	_____
12. Vision problems	_____	_____	_____
13. Hearing problems	_____	_____	_____
14. Alcohol	_____	_____	_____
15. Poor nutrition	_____	_____	_____

At this point, you might want to reread the information on the factors that pertain to you. Some of them may require professional treatment by a physician or counselor, while others can be lessened by changes in your environment or lifestyle. Almost everyone can improve memory skills by learning to use memory improvement techniques, so continue reading and consider which of the following techniques will be most useful in improving your memory.

EXERCISE: FACTORS THAT AFFECT MEMORY

True/False. Circle the answer.

T   F   1. Problems with vision or hearing can affect your memory.

T   F   2. Memory recall can be affected by emotional factors.

T   F   3. Poor memory is often due to poor observation.

T   F   4. Negative expectations have no effect on memory performance.

T   F   5. Memory problems rarely indicate the need to see a doctor.

T   F   6. Problems with your health can cause increased forgetting.

T   F   7. Only major stress will affect your memory.

T   F   8. Even if you're looking forward to a change of residence, you may notice some memory problems after you move.

T   F   9. Once your memory begins to get worse, it will never improve.

T   F   10. Increasing activity, through mental stimulation, social interaction, or physical exercise, may benefit memory.

See p. 96 for answers.

Appendix A: Alzheimer's Disease

The following material is reprinted by permission of the Alzheimer's Disease and Related Disorders Associated Inc., 919 North Michigan Avenue, Suite 1000, Chicago, Illinois 60611-1676.

What Is Alzheimer's Disease?

Alzheimer's disease (AD) is a progressive, degenerative disease that attacks the brain and results in impaired memory, thinking, and behavior. It affects an estimated 4 million American adults.

AD usually has a gradual onset. Problems remembering recent events and difficulty performing familiar tasks are early symptoms. Additionally, the Alzheimer patient may experience confusion, personality change, behavior change, impaired judgment, and difficulty finding words, finishing thoughts, or following directions. How quickly these changes occur will vary from person to person, but the disease eventually leaves its victims totally unable to care for themselves.

What Is the Difference between Alzheimer's and Senility?

Increasing public awareness of Alzheimer's disease and its devastating effects is causing many older adults and Alzheimer family members to fear that forgotten names or misplaced keys may be early signs of Alzheimer's.

Until recently, an older person who was forgetful and had difficulty caring for himself was labeled "senile." "Senility" was considered a normal part of aging.

The symptoms of "senility" are now described by the term "dementia." Health care professionals recognize that when memory loss interferes with daily activities, it is not normal and is most likely the result of a disease.

Dementia is not a normal part of aging. This is because its symptoms, which include difficulties with language, learning, thinking, and reasoning, as well as memory loss, eventually become severe enough to interfere with a person's work and social life.

Although Alzheimer's disease is the most common form of irreversible dementia, some forms of dementia are curable. Keep in mind, however, that the majority of adults over the age of 65 do not develop any form of dementia.

What Is "Normal" Memory Loss?

At some time, everyone forgets her keys or where the car is parked or the name of an acquaintance. Everyone forgets things as she goes about daily activities. Usually, we don't think anything of such brief memory lapses. Often, what has been forgotten is something of little importance and eventually the information is remembered.

Although most of us expect our bodies and our reflexes to slow down with age, physicians now recognize that many healthy individuals are also less able to remember certain types of information as they get older. Health care professionals use the term "age-associated memory impairment" (AAMI) to describe minor memory difficulties that come with age.

AAMI is neither progressive nor disabling, whereas some dementias are both. AAMI is often most noticeable when the individual is under pressure. Once the person is relaxed, he is able to remember the forgotten material without difficulty.

No "treatment" for age-associated memory loss has been developed. However, writing reminders and lists, repeating messages or names out loud, allowing more time to remember, and using association to remember names may be helpful.

In addition to AAMI, minor memory difficulties may be caused by distraction, fatigue, grief, depression, stress, illness, medication, alcohol, vision or hearing loss, lack of concentration, or an attempt to remember too many details at once.

In general, it may be beneficial to cut back on alcohol, eat well-balanced meals, and make sure that medications are being taken as prescribed and are not themselves causing problems.

Recognizing Dementia

How can you tell if memory loss is more serious than age-associated memory impairment?

Dementia is progressive. AAMI may remain unchanged for years.

Most individuals with AAMI can compensate for memory loss with reminders and notes. However, memory loss associated with dementia will begin to interfere with the normal activities of daily life. In addition, dementia will affect more than memory.

For instance, Alzheimer's disease affects the ability to use words, work with figures, solve problems, and use reasoning and judgment. Alzheimer's disease also may result in changes in mood and personality.

When "forgetfulness" starts to affect the ability to carry on daily activities, it is cause for concern. Even in advanced old age, memory loss that interferes with everyday life is not normal. It may indicate a form of dementia, and the individual should undergo a complete evaluation to find out the cause.

At this time, Alzheimer's disease cannot be cured. Related disorders such as multi-infarct dementia, Parkinson's disease, Huntington's disease, and Creutzfeldt-Jakob disease, also involve irreversible dementia.

Equally important to remember, though, are the many *reversible* causes of dementia—depression, nutritional and vitamin deficiencies, drug intoxication and interaction, thyroid imbalances, some infections, blood chemistry imbalances, tumors, some blood clots, normal pressure hydrocephalus, and excessive pressure in the brain from spinal fluid.

Getting a Diagnosis of Alzheimer's Disease

At this time, there is no single diagnostic test for Alzheimer's disease. To rule out other causes of dementia symptoms requires a complete medical, neurologic, and psychiatric evaluation, as well as neuropsychological tests. A complete history from the patient's family, including a description of the symptoms and progression, also is very valuable.

For more information on the symptoms of Alzheimer's and the necessary diagnostic tests, contact the Alzheimer's Association Chapter nearest you. The Chapter members may be able to refer you to appropriate local medical resources. Call the Association's toll-free number for the Chapter nearest you: 1-800-272-3900 (TDD: 312-335-8882).

What Is the Difference between AAMI and Alzheimer's Disease?

Activity	Alzheimer Patient	Age-Associated Memory Impairment Patient
Forgets	whole experience	parts of an experience
Remembers later	rarely	often
Follows written or spoken directions	gradually unable	usually able
Able to use notes	gradually unable	usually able
Able to care for self	gradually unable	usually able

Source: Derived from the book *Care of Alzheimer's Patients: A Manual for Nursing Home Staff,* by Lisa P. Gwyther.

Further Reading

Steps to Choosing a Physician, Action Series, Alzheimer's Association, 1991.

The 36-Hour Day: A Guide to Caring for Persons with Alzheimer's Disease and Related Dementing Illnesses, by Nancy L. Mace and Peter V. Rabins, M.D. Baltimore: Johns Hopkins University Press, 1991 (revised edition).

Understanding Alzheimer's Disease, edited by Miriam K. Aronson, Ed.D. New York: Scribner's, 1988.

All publications are available from the Alzheimer's Association national office and Chapters.

Appendix B: Nutrition

The following information is reprinted by permission of the Nutrition Screening Initiative, 2626 Pennsylvania Avenue N.W., Suite 301, Washington, DC 20037. The Nutrition Screening Initiative is a project of the American Academy of Family Physicians, the American Dietetic Association, and National Council on the Aging, Inc., and is funded in part by a grant from Ross Laboratories, a Division of Abbot Labs.

Determine Your Nutritional Health

The Warning Signs of poor nutritional health are often overlooked. Use this checklist to find out if you or someone you know is at nutritional risk. Read the statements below. Circle the number in the yes column for those that apply to you or someone you know. For each yes answer, score the number in the box. Total your nutritional score.

	Yes
I have an illness or condition that made me change the kind and/or amount of food I eat.	2
I eat fewer than 2 meals per day.	3
I eat few fruits or vegetables, or milk products.	2
I have 3 or more drinks of beer, liquor, or wine almost every day.	2
I have tooth or mouth problems that make it hard for me to eat.	2
I don't always have enough money to buy the food I need.	4
I eat alone most of the time.	1
I take 3 or more different prescribed or over-the-counter drugs a day.	1
Without wanting to, I have lost or gained 10 pounds in the last 6 months.	2
I am not always physically able to shop, cook and/or feed myself.	2

Total _____

Total Your Nutritional Score. If it's—

0–2 Good! Recheck your nutritional score in 6 months.

3–5 You are at moderate nutritional risk. See what can be done to improve your eating habits and lifestyle. Your office on aging, senior nutrition program, senior citizens center, or health department can help. Recheck your nutritional score in 3 months.

6 or more You are at high nutritional risk. Bring this checklist the next time you see your doctor, dietitian, or other qualified health or social service professional. Talk with them about any problems you may have. Ask for help to improve your nutritional health.

Remember that warning signs suggest risk, but do not represent diagnosis of any condition. Read on to learn more about the Warning Signs of poor nutritional health.

The Nutrition Checklist is based on the Warning Signs described below. Use the word *DETERMINE* to remind you of the Warning Signs.

DISEASE

Any disease, illness, or chronic condition which causes you to change the way you eat, or makes it hard for you to eat, puts your nutritional health at risk. Four out of five adults have chronic diseases that are affected by diet. Confusion or memory loss that keeps getting worse is estimated to affect one out of five or more of older adults. This can make it hard to remember what, when, or if you've eaten. Feeling sad or depressed, which happens to about one in eight older adults, can cause big changes in appetite, digestion, energy level, weight, and well-being.

EATING POORLY

Eating too little and eating too much both lead to poor health. Eating the same foods day after day or not eating fruit, vegetables, and milk products daily will also cause poor nutritional health. One in five adults skips meals daily. Only 13% of adults eat the minimum amount of fruit and vegetables needed. One in four older adults drinks too much alcohol. Many health problems become worse if you drink more than one or two alcoholic beverages per day.

TOOTH LOSS/MOUTH PAIN

A healthy mouth, teeth, and gums are needed to eat. Missing, loose, or rotten teeth or dentures which don't fit well or cause mouth sores make it hard to eat.

ECONOMIC HARDSHIP

As many as 40% of older Americans have incomes of less than $6,000 per year. Having less—or choosing to spend less—than $25–30 per week for food makes it very hard to get the foods you need to stay healthy.

REDUCED SOCIAL CONTACT

One-third of all older people live alone. Being with people daily has a positive effect on morale, well-being, and eating.

MULTIPLE MEDICINES

Many older Americans must take medicines for health problems. Almost half of older Americans take multiple medicines daily. Growing old may change the way we respond to drugs. The more medicines you take, the greater the chance for side effects such as increased or decreased appetite, change in taste, constipation, weakness, drowsiness, diarrhea, nausea, and others. Vitamins or minerals when taken in large doses act like drugs and can cause harm. Alert your doctor to everything you take.

INVOLUNTARY WEIGHT LOSS/GAIN

Losing or gaining a lot of weight when you are not trying to do so is an important warning sign that must not be ignored. Being overweight or underweight also increases your chance of poor health.

NEEDS ASSISTANCE IN SELF CARE

Although most older people are able to eat, one of every five has trouble walking, shopping, and buying and cooking food, especially as they get older.

ELDER YEARS ABOVE AGE 80

Most older people lead full and productive lives. But as age increases, risk of frailty and health problems increases. Checking your nutritional health regularly makes good sense.

4 Memory Improvement Techniques

Everyone has to make choices about what is important to remember. No one remembers everything. Once you have determined that you want to improve your memory in a particular area, you can select a strategy for change. In this chapter we describe sixteen techniques for improving your memory. They are:

- association
- visualization
- active observation
- elaboration
- written reminders
- auditory reminders
- environmental change
- self-instruction
- story method
- chunking
- first letter cues
- create a word
- categorization
- search your memory
- alphabet search
- review

Some of these techniques involve cues in your environment, such as notes, lists, signs, or buzzers. Other techniques improve the way you encode the information you want to remember so that you can retrieve it more easily. Some of these techniques will be familiar; others will seem strange. It is difficult to know which ones will be useful for you without trying them several times. Look for chances to experiment.

We have found that it is fun and rewarding to figure out a way to remember and to succeed. We believe that there is a tool for remembering almost anything. However, in some cases you may decide that the effort needed is not worth the benefit gained. Recognize that the choice is yours to make.

Here's the best way to use these memory improvement techniques:

1. Choose something specific that you want to remember.
2. Review the possible techniques and select one.
3. Try the technique. (If it works, congratulations!)
4. If your chosen technique does not work, try something else.
5. Don't feel defeated if some things are particularly hard to remember. Ask yourself if it really matters anyway.

WHAT ARE SOME GENERAL STRATEGIES FOR IMPROVING MEMORY?

Although there are many techniques for remembering specific kinds of information, there are four strategies that can be used whenever you want to encode almost any kind of new information securely so that it is available for retrieval.

The four general strategies for improving memory are:

Association: Associate what you want to remember with what you know.

Visualization: Visualize a picture of what you want to remember.

Active observation: Actively observe and think about what you want to remember.

Elaboration: Elaborate on the details of the information you want to remember.

People who have excellent memories use these strategies on a daily basis. It will take thought and practice, but if you can incorporate these strategies into everyday life, you will have a better memory.

Associate What You Want to Remember with What You Know

Association is the process of forming mental connections between what you want to remember and what you already know. Although many associations are made automatically, the conscious creation of associations is an excellent strategy for encoding new information. Once you make an association, repeating it several times either in your head or aloud will help you remember.

This technique can be used to remember:

- the name of your new neighbor
- the street where your friend lives
- the title of a movie you want to recommend
- whether to turn right or left to get to the restaurant
- the number of the bus to your friend's house

EXAMPLES

- *Mr. Miller:* My daughter asked me to pick up a special kind of crackers called Cheese Delight at the grocery store. I wanted to see if I could remember it without writing it down, so I worked on figuring out an association. Crackers and cheese have always been a good combination to me, so I could remember the "cheese" part easily. The "delight" part was a little more difficult. I thought about how delighted I would be if I could succeed at this task and registered the word and feeling in my mind. When I got to the store and looked at the countless kinds of crackers, the Cheese Delight box jumped right out at me and I thought, "Association really works!"

- *Mr. Cavender:* I have two cars that have gas caps on opposite sides, and I could never remember which was which. Each time I went to fill up, I had to ponder which way to approach the gas pumps, and I felt aggravated. I decided to consciously find an association that would register the information once and for all. I first noted that the gas cap was on the left side of my tan car. Now, what could I associate with left? I thought about the fact that this car is lighter in color than my black car, so I could associate the "l" in *light* and *left*. For several weeks, each time I drove into the gas station, I said to myself, "In this light car, the gas cap is on the left."

- *Ms. Spencer:* I had a new neighbor whose name was Marsha. For some reason I had a hard time remembering her name. I had learned about association in a memory course and decided to try it. After looking carefully at Marsha, I noticed she had white, fluffy hair. I decided that I could remember her name by associating Marsha with marshmallow. Each time I saw her, I associated her hair with a big marshmallow and said to myself, "Marshmallow Marsha."

EXERCISE: ASSOCIATION

Create an association between the following items of new information and something you already know.

1. You must remember to take the entrance marked "west" on the expressway to get to the doctor's office.

_____

_____

_____

2. You want to remember the year your grandson was born, which is 1968.

_____

_____

_____

3. You want to remember Rose Campbell's name.

_____

_____

_____

4. You want to remember the name "Turner Medical Clinic."

_____

_____

_____

See p. 96 for possible answers.

Visualize a Picture of What You Want to Remember

You have often heard that a picture is worth a thousand words. Visualization is the process of consciously creating an image in your mind of a task, a number, a name, a word, or an abstract thought. If you take the time to translate words into a meaningful picture and hold that picture in your mind for a few seconds, you are more likely to remember the name, the task, or the thought.

This technique can be used to remember:

- items you need to buy at the grocery store
- the route from the airport terminal to where you parked your car
- the laundry basket you want to bring up from the basement
- the name of a new breakfast cereal that you want to try
- the punch line of a joke you recently heard

EXAMPLES

- *Mrs. Pinelle:* When I was shopping last month, I saw such a beautiful dress in the window of a new store called Toshiros. I knew I'd never remember the name of this shop because it was unfamiliar to me, and I didn't know what it meant. When I repeated the name over to myself, I imagined a big hairy toe and a razor getting ready to shear the hair off—"Toe-shear-o."

- *Ms. Barton:* I love to tell my friends about my favorite restaurant. It's so expensive that I can only go there once a year, so I don't see the name very often. It's called Justine's, which is a name I have trouble remembering. However, I do know that they have a young chef, so I imagine a very youthful face with a big chef's hat on, and think "Why, he's 'just a teen.'"

- *Mr. Simon:* I get so angry when I get up from my chair, put on my coat, walk to the back of my yard to get something from the garage, then forget what I went to get. After taking a memory course, I found out that if I take the time to picture what I'm getting up for, I can remember most of the time. Just yesterday, I wanted the flashlight from my car. I remembered it as blue, and I envisioned myself using it to look in the attic. When I got to the car, I had no trouble remembering what I went for.

EXERCISE: VISUALIZATION

Create a visual image to help you remember the following:

1. Mrs. Hammerman's name

_____

_____

_____

2. An echogram

_____

_____

_____

3. Parkinson's disease

_____

_____

_____

4. Lane 5B in a parking lot

_____

_____

_____

5. To buy a new windshield wiper blade while at the gas station

_____

_____

_____

See page 97 for possible answers.

Actively Observe and Think about What You Want to Remember

It is often difficult to remember things that you haven't observed clearly or with much interest. Active observation is the process of consciously paying attention to the details of what you see, hear, or read. By using active observation you can find meaning and vibrancy in a photograph, a new face, a nature scene, a conversation, an occurrence on the street, or a piece of artwork. Active observation contrasts with a passive attitude of letting life go on around you without much thought or interest. To actively observe a subject, think about the meaning of the subject, how you feel about it, how it affects you, and whether you *want* to remember it. Ask yourself questions that will reinforce its meaning. One key to remembering is being interested.

This technique can be used to remember:

- the design of a quilt you saw in a store
- how to play a new game that your grandchild is teaching you
- the faces of people you see in the hallway of your apartment complex
- the difference between a fir tree and a juniper

EXAMPLES

- *Mrs. Sung:* I have very bad arthritis and am in a wheelchair. I was so depressed and bored—every day was just the same, and my memory was getting really bad. My daughter gave me a bird feeder for my birthday, and little by little I started watching the birds that came. One day I saw a bird I didn't recognize. I asked my daughter if she knew what it was. She didn't, either, but the next time she visited me, she brought a colored picture book of hundreds of birds and facts about them. When we looked up the bird, I was amazed at how many kinds there are in Michigan. That bird feeder has changed my life! I'm seeing and learning new things, and I'm surprised that I can really remember them.

- *Miss Robinson:* I parked in a large parking garage when going to Senior Power Day at the state capitol building. There were several up and down ramps on each level and no letters or numbers designating the area in which I parked. I realized that I could easily misplace my car. I carefully observed the route I took to the exit stairway and, when I got there, looked back to reinforce the image of the location of my car. When I returned several hours later, I had a strong memory of where my car was located and how to get there.

- *Mr. Hooper:* After taking a memory course and learning about active observation, I decided to give it a try. I went to our local museum and spent some time looking at a painting of two women by Monet. Instead of just glancing at the painting as I usually do, I looked at the details as well as the whole and asked myself some questions: Did I think it was pretty? What time of year was it? Did the women look happy or sad? What were they wearing? Was there anything especially unusual about the painting? Would I like to have it in my living room? When I left the museum, I knew that I would remember something from this trip to the museum; it would not be just the usual blur of pictures.

EXERCISE: ACTIVE OBSERVATION

Look at the picture below, consciously paying attention to the details. Ask yourself questions about the picture's meaning and its effect on you as you look at it.

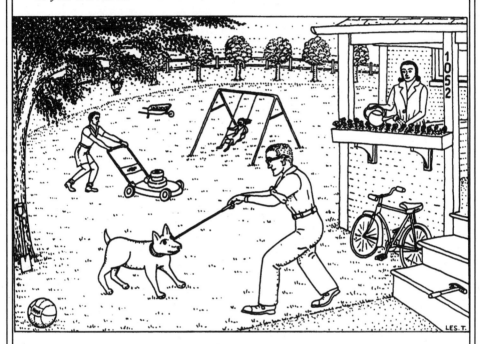

Now, cover the picture and see if you can answer these questions.

- How many people are in the picture?
- What is the boy doing?
- What is the woman doing?
- What is leaning against the house?
- What is on the steps?
- Name the items in the yard.
- What is the number on the house?
- What is the boy wearing?
- What is the man doing?

If you are able to answer all of the above questions, you have used excellent powers of observation. Take a second look, if you aren't sure of the correct answers.

Elaborate on the Details of the Information
You Want to Remember

A brief, unexamined thought is very fragile and easily forgotten. When we elaborate on the details of a thought or idea, we encode it more deeply. We experience this depth of processing unintentionally when something very interesting or controversial occurs. In our minds, we comment on the occurrence; we try to understand what happened; we relate it to what we know of the situation; we ask ourselves how we feel about it. This process can be used intentionally as a strategy for encoding information we want to remember.

Try this technique if you want to remember:

- the instructions for using your new vacuum attachments
- the platforms of the two mayoral candidates
- the courses that your grandson is taking in college
- the directions to the new recreation building.

EXAMPLES

- *Mr. Simon:* I recently purchased a new VCR, read the instructions, and tediously followed them to record my favorite TV show. The next time I tried to record a show, I couldn't remember what to do and had to reread the instruction manual. Because I wanted to be able to program my VCR in the future without referring to the manual, I was determined to encode the information well by using the technique of elaboration. I talked myself through the steps, figuring out the order and importance of each step. I translated the stilted manual directions into my own language. I repeated the steps several times to fix them in my long-term memory. I discovered that it works even better if you use this technique aloud. Even after being on vacation for three weeks, I could still remember the steps.

- *Miss Kirby:* I took a trip of a lifetime to the Hawaiian Islands. I visited three of the islands—all of which are gorgeous, yet different from each other. I wanted to be able to tell my friends about the islands without mixing them up. I had read in the newspaper that if you elaborate on the details of what you want to remember, you will encode the information more deeply. I thought about the different physical characteristics of the island, what I did on each island, and where I stayed. I made some associations between these details and the names of the islands. For several days I repeated these details, and now I find it easy to remember.

EXERCISE: ELABORATION

Every state has a nickname by which it is known. Here are the nicknames of three states:

Minnesota: The Gopher State
Missouri: The Show Me State
Montana: The Treasure State

See if you can use elaboration to encode these states and their nicknames so that you can remember them tomorrow. When you wake up tomorrow, ask yourself if you can remember this information. If not, try elaborating on it more fully.

DO I HAVE TO REMEMBER EVERYTHING IN MY HEAD?

Although there are times when you have to rely upon your mind for remembering, most of us use external reminders to prompt us throughout our daily lives. For example, we may use an alarm clock to wake up in the morning; keep a calendar of appointments; make grocery lists; use a kitchen timer for baking cookies; and use a marked pill box. Everyone agrees that there is no need to trust our memory in these situations. If we can use something in our environment to cue us, our minds are free to think of other things. Even though the following three external techniques may be familiar to you, consider finding new ways to adapt them to your needs:

Written reminders: Write things down.

Auditory reminders: Use sound to trigger your memory.

Environmental change: Change something in your surroundings so that it jogs your memory.

Write Things Down

Although people of all ages use lists, calendars, appointment books, and notes to keep track of what they want to remember, many older people believe that written reminders shouldn't be necessary. Writing things down is one of the most useful memory tools. As you age you may need to make even greater use of written reminders for both future events and as a diary of the day's happenings.

If you are having trouble remembering the people you meet, what you read, or how you spend your day, keep all that information in one diary. On a similar note, all financial papers and bills should be kept in one place and recorded systematically.

EXAMPLES

- Keep a running list of things you need to do. As soon as you think of something, add it to the list. Keep this list in a permanent place where you can't help but notice it.

- Use an appointment book or calendar to remind yourself of upcoming events and make a habit of looking at it frequently.

- Keep a list of health questions you want to ask your physician at your next appointment. Write down instructions from the physician before you leave the office.

- Keep a diary of what has happened each day so that if you wonder whether you've written a letter or made an important phone call you can refer to the diary. Include the names of people you've met.

- Keep a list of books you want to read or have read.

- Keep a notebook where you record letters and greeting cards sent and received.

 ASSIGNMENT

Within the next three days buy a notebook that you will use to record whatever you want to remember. Keep a record for one week.

For example:

Pd. car insurance
sent package to Jane
met new neighbor —Jack

Buy thread
Call plumber 769-1130
Watch TV special
on S. Africa   9:00

Use Sound to Trigger Your Memory

Alarm clocks and kitchen timers can be used to remind yourself of something that can't be done immediately but that must be done at a specific time. A telephone answering machine can also be used to provide an auditory cue.

EXAMPLES

- If you make a phone call and get a busy signal, set your kitchen timer to remind yourself to call again.

- If you're busy writing letters and want to be sure to leave for an appointment at a specific time, set the kitchen timer and carry it with you to your desk.

- If you are away from home and want to remember to do something when you return, leave yourself a message on your answering machine.

Change Something in Your Surroundings So That It Jogs Your Memory

One of the best and easiest ways to remind yourself of a specific task is to change something in your environment so that you notice the change. It then serves as a cue to jog your memory. It is imperative that you make the change as soon as you think of the task.

EXAMPLES

- Put the clothes to take to the cleaners in front of the door.

- Move the telephone out of its ordinary place as a way to remind yourself to call someone later.

- Put a note on the refrigerator so that you'll see it when you eat breakfast and remember to send a card to your son.

- Put a note on the steering wheel to remind yourself to vote or stop at the cleaners.

- Tie a string around the handles of your purse so that you can't open it without being reminded of what you need to do.

- Put an empty box in front of the basement stairway to remind yourself to turn off the electric heater when you go upstairs.

- Change your watch or ring to the other hand; you will constantly feel it, and it will remind you of what you need to do.

When using any of these external reminders, it is crucial to avoid procrastination. As soon as you think of something you need to do in the future, choose one of these techniques and act upon it. If you think, "I'll add potatoes to my grocery list when this TV show is over," you may forget all about it ten minutes later.

EXERCISE: ENVIRONMENTAL CHANGE
Think of ways to jog your memory for the following tasks by using environmental change.

1. You want to remember to bring your lasagna pan to the senior center tomorrow.

   _____

   _____

   _____

   _____

   _____

2. You are out grocery shopping and want to remember to call your dentist when you get home.

_____

_____

_____

_____

3. You are at your exercise class and a friend asks you to bring a certain book to tomorrow's class.

_____

_____

_____

_____

4. You want to remember to put out the garbage tomorrow.

_____

_____

_____

_____

5. You are sitting in church and you remember that you have to stop at the store on your way home.

_____

_____

_____

_____

See p. 97 for possible solutions.

HOW CAN I AVOID WORRYING ABOUT WHETHER I HAVE DONE WHAT I INTENDED TO DO?

Many daily tasks are done automatically; we don't pay much attention to them. In order to avoid worrying about whether you have unplugged the iron, turned off the electric blanket, or locked the door, you can use the technique of *self-instruction.*

Give Yourself Verbal Instructions about What You Want to Remember

Self-instruction is the process of giving yourself mental or verbal reinforcement so that you will pay attention to what you want to remember. This technique is powerful because it focuses your attention on an act that is often done automatically and thus is easily forgotten. Use this technique to fix in your mind tasks about which you may ask yourself later, "Did I remember to do that?" As you turn off the coffeepot, say aloud to yourself, "I am now turning off the coffeepot," and you won't wonder about it later.

Sometimes you can use this technique to remind yourself to do something in the immediate future. You might need to provide more detail to reinforce your memory for a future task. As you drive to the grocery store at dusk, remind yourself aloud to turn off the lights. One sentence is not enough in this case. You might say, "I'm putting my lights on as I go to the grocery store. When I get into the parking lot at Supermart, I must remember to turn them off." You might also visualize the lights shining on the store window as you arrive, then see yourself turning them off.

EXAMPLE

- *Ms. Heinz:* One thing I hoped to get out of a memory course was learning how to remember whether I put detergent in the washer. I would get upstairs and have to go back down because I was never sure whether I did it. The instructors suggested that, as I add the detergent, I say to myself, "There, I just put the soap into the washer." I gave it a try, and now I always say something aloud like, "Good, I won't have to come down here again because I just added the soap," and it really works for me.

 ASSIGNMENT ————————————————————————

For the rest of the day, use self-instruction whenever you perform a task that might cause you to ask later, "Did I do that?" At the end of the day look through the list below and check the ways you used this technique or might use it in the future. Notice if using this technique was helpful.

- turning off the stove/iron/coffeepot/heater
- locking the door
- turning off the car lights
- turning down the heat
- adding the laundry soap
- making a phone call
- taking medicine
- turning off the basement light/front porch light
- closing the garage door
- putting the gas cap back on the gas tank
- watering the plants
- other

ARE THERE ANY TECHNIQUES THAT COULD HELP WHEN I HAVE SEVERAL ITEMS TO REMEMBER?

It is always easier to remember fewer items than more. Look for ways to connect or combine the items so that they can be remembered collectively. You'll understand this concept when you read about the following techniques:

Story method: Devise a story that will connect things you want to remember.

Chunking: Chunk individual items into a group.

First letter cues: Group the first letters of a series of items.

Create a word: Expand random letters into a familiar word.

Categorization: Group a list of items by category.

Devise a Story That Will Connect Things You Want to Remember

The story method is the process of making up a simple, yet colorful, tale connecting items that seem to have no connection. This is a technique that many people resist because it seems either silly or too complicated. We believe that if you give it a try, you will find it amazingly effective. This technique can be used to remember:

- two phone calls that you need to make when you get home
- three things you want to tell your daughter when you call her
- three items you need to pick up at the hardware store
- two books you want to get at the library.

─── EXAMPLES ───

- You wake up in the night and start thinking of what you need to do the next day. You want to remember that you need to call your dentist, return a rug to the department store, and get an oil change for your car, but you don't want to get out of bed to make a list.

You make up a story connecting these items by visualizing your dentist using a rug to keep himself warm because his car has run out of oil and is stalled.

• You think of four items that you want to buy at the drugstore: a birthday card, a sponge, a bottle of shampoo, and some film. You create a story about shampooing your hair with a sponge while signing a birthday card, and a photographer bursts in to take your photo.

EXERCISE: STORY METHOD

Make up a one- or two-sentence story connecting the following items:

1. Getting a duplicate key made, picking up a birthday cake, and going to the bank

_____

_____

_____

_____

_____

2. Shopping for stationery, cologne, and a broom

_____

_____

_____

_____

_____

See p. 97 for possible solutions.

Chunk Individual Items into a Group

It is easier to remember three items than seven. When you are trying to remember a group of numbers, look for ways to combine them. This technique can be used to remember:

- phone numbers
- street addresses and zip codes
- social security and driver's license numbers

EXAMPLES

- If you want to remember a local telephone number such as 764-2556, you can usually remember the prefix because it is fairly familiar. However, if you group the last four numbers into two chunks, 25 and 56, the phone number will be easier to recall.

- A driver's license or social security number may seem almost impossible to remember. However, if you learn it in chunks it will be more manageable. 343–49–4296 could be 3-43-49-42-96 or 34-34-94-29-6 or 343-494-296.

EXERCISE: CHUNKING

Memorize your driver's license number or Social Security number by chunking the individual numbers. Analyze the sequence to see which way of chunking makes the most sense.

_____

_____

_____

Group the First Letters of a Series of Items

This technique involves using the first letters of a list of words to form either another word or a meaningful sentence whose words begin with the same letters as the words on the list. Although this technique is hard to describe, it's easy to use. The following examples should give you the idea.

EXAMPLES

- If you want to remember the names of the five Great Lakes, you can take the first letter of each lake and create the word HOMES (Huron, Ontario, Michigan, Erie, Superior).

- If you want to remember the names of each of the presidents from Eisenhower to Clinton, you can take the first letter of each name and form a sentence that has meaning to you. One example is: "Every kid juggles nine fine china rings before class" (Eisenhower, Kennedy, Johnson, Nixon, Ford, Carter, Reagan, Bush, Clinton).

- You are in your car and think of four items you want from the grocery store and have no paper to write them on. You need butter, apples, lemon, and milk. By rearranging the first letters of these four items, you find that you can form the word "lamb," which will serve as a memory cue. If the items do not form a word, try making a sentence with matching first letters. For example, if your list is soup, chicken, soap, and lettuce, you could create the sentence "Some cooks like soup."

EXERCISE: FIRST LETTER CUES

1. *Create a word or sentence out of the first letters of the names of these downtown streets to help you remember the order. In this case, it's important to keep the letters in the same order as the streets.*

   Main

   Adams

   Lincoln

   Rose

   Brown

   _____

   _____

   _____

   _____

2. *Try using this technique to remember the names of your cousin's children.*

   Rob

   Alice

   Chris

   _____

   _____

   _____

   _____

See p. 97 for possible solutions.

Expand Random Letters into a Familiar Word

Sometimes you need to remember a group of letters that make no inherent sense, for example, license plates or business names. In this case you can add more letters, often vowels, to form a familiar word.

EXAMPLES

- On a license plate, you might make the word "extra" out of "xra" or "lefty" out of "lft."

- If you have trouble remembering the name of the company that manages your apartment building, PND, expand these letters to form the word *panda*.

EXERCISE: CREATE A WORD
Expand the following letters into words:

1. PLM _____

2. RBT _____

3. GLW _____

4. STR _____

5. HLD _____

See p. 98 for possible solutions.

Group a List of Items by Category

Categorization is the process of looking at a random list of items and seeing how to group them by category. It is easier to remember three categories that serve as cues for the nine items in the list than to remember each of the nine items separately.

EXAMPLES

• The following nine items could be grouped into three categories:

popcorn	tuna	chips	applesauce	cookies
peas	milk	juice	pop	

Canned goods: peas applesauce tuna

Snacks: popcorn chips cookies

Liquids: milk juice pop

EXERCISE: CATEGORIZATION
Categorize the following items:

Windex	broom	paper towels
Scotch tape	envelopes	dish soap
glue	sponge	furniture polish
bleach		

_____

_____

_____

_____

_____

See p. 98 for possible solutions.

IS THERE ANYTHING THAT WILL HELP ME RECALL
WELL-KNOWN INFORMATION WHEN I NEED IT?

When you know that the information you desire is in your long-term memory but you can't retrieve it when you want it, there are three techniques that you will find helpful:

- *Search your memory:* Search your memory bank for related facts that may serve as cues.
- *Alphabet search:* Go through the alphabet to jog your memory.
- *Review:* Review in advance what you may be called upon to remember.

Search Your Memory Bank for Related Facts
That May Serve as Cues

When you can't think of something that you know is in your long-term memory, merely thinking longer and harder often does not work. However, there is a technique that is often useful. When you want to retrieve specific information from long-term memory, try thinking of related facts that serve as cues to trigger the information you are looking for.

This technique can be used for recalling:

- the name of a famous person
- the French word for *friend*
- the name of a TV show
- how to get somewhere that you haven't been for a long time
- the state in which the Grand Canyon is located.

EXAMPLES

- *Ms. Scott:* I met a woman at a party last week. When she introduced herself, I knew I had met her before. I remembered our interaction clearly, but I couldn't remember at whose home we had met. After I left the party, I searched for cues related to our initial meeting that would trigger the information about where we met. I thought about our conversation, how long ago the initial meeting took place, other people involved in the conversation, and my feelings about the interaction. It suddenly occurred to me that we had met earlier at a party given by a co-worker.

- *Mrs. McFadden:* My daughter lives in a new subdivision in town that has a special name, which I have trouble remembering. I wanted to tell my neighbor, but I didn't want to bother my daughter at work. I thought, "Maybe if I think of some related information, it will help." I could remember my daughter's address: 272 Appomattox. I thought about the entry sign to the subdivision that has a cannon on it. "It must have something to do with the Civil War." It came to me—Gettysburg!

EXERCISE: SEARCH YOUR MEMORY
See if you can recall the two candidates who ran for president of the United States in 1980. If you don't immediately know, search your memory for related facts that could serve as cues for this information.

_____

_____

See p. 98 for the answer.

Go through the Alphabet to Jog Your Memory

Alphabet search is the process of thinking through the sounds of the letters of the alphabet from *A* to *Z* to see if one will serve as a cue to jog your memory.

EXAMPLES

- If you're trying to remember the name of someone you have just met, run through the sounds of the alphabet. Hearing the sound of the letter *m* may trigger the name Marian.

- You want to describe the food you ate last night to a friend but can't remember the word *fettucine*. You might go through the alphabet hoping that the beginning sound of one of the letters will cue your memory.

Is there anything you can do to optimize your chances of remembering familiar names?

When you know in advance that you will be called upon to use the names of familiar persons, places, or things, you can use the following technique to prepare.

**Review in Advance What You May
Be Called upon to Remember**

Everyone knows the feeling of forgetting familiar information, such as a friend's name or a well-known author. When you have to recall this type of information on demand, it sometimes takes a few seconds to bring it to mind—just long enough to cause a mental block. This experience is especially likely to happen if you are asked to recall something or someone you haven't thought about for a while. When you *know* you will be called upon to remember certain names or information, reviewing ahead of time will often eliminate this problem.

This technique can be used to help you keep in mind:

- the names of the grandnieces and grandnephews you will be seeing tomorrow
- the history of your medical problems when you see your doctor
- things you want to ask your grandchild when you take him out to lunch
- the names of people you will be seeing at the annual meeting of your condominium association

---

EXAMPLES

- If you are going to a family reunion or church social and are afraid you will not remember everyone's name, prepare ahead of time by going over a list of all who might attend. Writing down the names and saying them aloud is more effective than simply reading through a list. As you say the name, visualize the person and something special about him or her, like red hair or a great laugh.

- If you are going to a meeting of your book club, record the title of the book, the author, the names of characters, and your feelings about the book and review them before you go.

- If you are going to lunch with a friend, review the names of your friend's children and what you know about them beforehand so that you can talk about them easily.

EXERCISE: REVIEW

Think of the next group meeting that you will attend (exercise class, senior center lunch group, bridge club, temple group) or try to think of the names of the people who live near you. List the names below and review them several times. If you have trouble listing all of them at one time, add to the list as the names come to you.

_____

_____

_____

_____

_____

_____

_____

_____

_____

Did review help you remember the names more easily?

General Tips for Remembering

1. **Believe in yourself.** Don't let negative expectations defeat you. If you expect to fail, you won't even try. If you find yourself thinking, "I can't remember names," substitute "I may forget some names, but by using memory improvement techniques I can do better."

2. **Make conscious choices about what you want to remember.** No one can remember everything. So put effort and energy into those areas that are most important to you.

3. **Focus your attention on what you really want to remember.** Much of what is called forgetting is a lack of attention. Before you blame your memory, ask yourself if you were really paying attention.

4. **Cut out distractions.** Keep in mind that as you age, you may find it more difficult to pay attention to more than one thing at a time. Recognize the limitations of short-term memory and cut out distractions whenever possible.

5. **Give yourself plenty of time.** People of all ages forget more frequently when they are rushing. In general, if you have enough time to think about what you need to accomplish, you are less

likely to forget something. You may also find that you need more time for learning new information and for recalling information from long-term memory. Give yourself a little additional time and see if it helps in encoding and retrieving information.

6. **Use all of your senses.** Use as many senses as possible when you want to remember something well. When you say something aloud, you hear the sound. When you write something down, you see the words. If you want to remember the size or shape of something, use your sense of touch. Smell and taste are very powerful in triggering memories from long ago.

7. **Be organized.** The old saying, "A place for everything, and everything in its place" is good advice for memory improvement. Make a decision to improve your organizational skills in whatever ways are important to you. If you routinely put your keys, glasses, purse, and bills in the same place, you will not waste time searching for them.

8. **Recognize and deal with the factors that may be negatively affecting your memory.** Certain factors can affect the memory process for people of all ages, but as you grow older, you may experience more of these negative influences. Think about which factors might be affecting your memory and look for possible solutions or ways to compensate.

9. **Relax.** Tension interferes with the memory process; relaxing often lets the memory come to the surface. When you feel anxious about the possibility of forgetting, you may become preoccupied with the anxiety and unable to concentrate on recalling the needed information. The solution is to take a deep breath and relax; frequently the information will come to you.

10. **Laugh.** Laughter breaks the tension of forgetting and keeps a memory lapse in perspective. When you start to tell a friend about a book that you are reading and can't remember the title, or begin to introduce your niece and can't come up with her name, admit that the word or name just escaped your mind, and laugh. Everyone has had that experience and can empathize.

11. **Enjoy past memories.** Recognize the richness of your storehouse of memories. You can experience great pleasure from recalling the events and people that have made up the fabric of your life. Life review can put the past and present into perspective. Take pride in your ability to remember the past and make it come alive for yourself and others.

Answers to the Exercises

Recall (p. 10) **and Recognition** (p. 13)

1. Dogpatch
2. Judy Garland
3. Iwo Jima
4. Spiro Agnew

Understanding the Memory Process (pp. 14–15)

When you go to the library and notice that there are a lot of colorful books on the "new books" shelf, you are using *sensory memory.* You read through the titles and think about whether they interest you. These conscious thoughts occur in *short-term memory.* Then you notice a book by a favorite author, James Michener. You take down the book, notice how long it is, read the dust jacket, and decide that you don't have time to read it this month. This process is called *encoding.* The information about the book leaves your conscious thought and goes into *long-term memory,* where it may be available for *retrieval* at another time. When you get home, you notice another of Michener's books in your den. This favorite book serves as a *cue* and reminds you of the book in the library. The connection between the library book and your book is called *association.*

How Memory Works (p. 16)

1. F	5. T
2. F	6. T
3. T	7. F
4. T	

Learning New Information (pp. 21–22)

1. Who and how many people you know
2. High motivation; low number of major life changes
3. Yes
4. It's important for older job seekers to get connected

How Memory Changes (p. 25)

1. F	4. T
2. F	5. F
3. T	6. T

Factors That Affect Memory (p. 50)

1. T	6. T
2. T	7. F
3. T	8. T
4. F	9. F
5. F	10. T

Association (p. 63)

1. Since you are going to the doctor, associate *west* with *wellness*.
2. Associate 1968 with the fact that the Tigers won the pennant that year, and you think of your grandson as a winner.
3. Associate *Campbell* with Campbell's soup and *Rose* with the red of the label on the soup can.
4. Associate the name *Turner* with turning your health around. Say to yourself several times, "Turner turned my health around."

Visualization (pp. 65–66)

1. Visualize a giant hammer hitting a man.
2. Imagine a tunnel with the sound of a heartbeat bouncing off the walls and echoing over and over.
3. Visualize a woman sitting in the park with the sun beating down on her shoulders.
4. Visualize five Balloons tied to your car antenna.
5. Visualize yourself paying for a tank of gas and asking the attendant for a replacement windshield wiper.

Environmental Change (pp. 74–75)

1. Put the pan in front of the door as soon as you think about bringing it.
2. Write yourself a note on the grocery bag in big letters so that when you unpack the groceries you'll see it.
3. Tie a string around your purse handle or wrist. When you get home you will be reminded to get the book out. Be sure to put it with your exercise clothes or equipment.
4. Put a big sign on the refrigerator or front door.
5. Change your watch or ring to the other hand.

Story Method (p. 79)

1. Envision a birthday cake shaped like a safe. You use a key to open it and find a huge pile of money.
2. See yourself breaking the bottle of cologne and sweeping up the pieces into a box of stationery.

First Letter Cues (p. 82)

1. Mother Always Liked Rose Best.
2. CAR or ARC

Create a Word (p. 83)

1. plum
2. robot
3. glow
4. string
5. hold

Categorization (p. 84)

Desk items	Utensils	Cleaning products
envelopes	sponge	Windex
Scotch tape	broom	dish soap
glue	paper towels	furniture polish
		bleach

Search Your Memory (p. 86)

Jimmy Carter and Ronald Reagan

Recommended Reading

Alan Baddeley. *Your Memory: A User's Guide*. New York: Macmillan, 1982.

Kathleen Gose and Gloria Levi. *Dealing with Memory Changes as You Grow Older*. New York: Bantam Books, 1988.

Danielle C. Lapp. *Don't Forget*. New York: McGraw-Hill, 1987.

Joan Minninger. *Total Recall*. New York: Pocket Books, 1984.

Edith Nalle Schafer. *Our Remarkable Memory*. Washington, D.C.: Starhill Press, 1988.

Robin West. *Memory Fitness over Forty*. Gainesville, Fla.: Triad Publications, 1985.

Library of Congress Cataloging-in-Publication Data

Fogler, Janet.
   Improving your memory : how to remember what you're starting to forget / Janet
Fogler and Lynn Stern — Rev. ed.
       p.   cm.
   Includes bibliographical references.
   ISBN 0-8018-4768-0 (pbk. : alk. paper)
   1. Memory in old age.   2. Memory—Age factors.   3. Mnemonics.   I. Stern, Lynn,
1949–   . II. Title.
BF724.85.M45F64   1994
153.1'2'0846—dc20   93-36782